The Fighter's Way

Muay Thai Handbook

Mr Nick Gorman

ISBN : 1500454702
ISBN 13: 9781500454708

Author's Note

A special thanks goes out to all those who have been a part of my fighting life, from the days with Quentin Chong at Dragon Power Gym to the South African team to the IFMA World Championships in 2007 and 2008. Thanks also to the Black Hawks for the brief stint in Johannesburg. Thank you to all my students, coaches, training partners, and those I have climbed into the ring with; you have all inspired me in some way.

Thank you to my family for the support over the years—my brothers and my mom, my mascot who is always in my corner. Lastly, to my late father, thank you for giving me the opportunities I've had; I take you with me everywhere I go. This book is a tribute to you.

This has been an incredible journey, and I'm so grateful to those who have been a part of it.

Nick Gorman

one

The Beginning

When I was nineteen years old, I climbed a mountain in Wales and gave my mother a call. I told her I was unhappy, and I wanted to change. I had just finished school and went on a gap year to work abroad in the United Kingdom. It was an invaluable experience, but I felt empty. It's quite hard for me to explain this emptiness, but I knew there had to be more to life than what I was experiencing. We all have our different desires and passions, but something was lacking. I undervalued myself. I thought I should be doing more, but I wasn't, and so this brought me down.

At this point I wanted to join the British army, and I told my parents that. The wise words from my father were to come back home and get a degree. He wasn't too concerned about what I studied, but he emphasized that I must study and get a degree. My father always had the amazing ability to step in when I needed him and give me direction.

I returned to my home in Cape Town, South Africa. My brother and some friends had taken up a martial art called Muay Thai, or "The Art of Eight Limbs," after the way you transform your hands, elbows, legs, and knees into an eight-in-one weapon. It is renowned as the world's most brutal ring sport, and it is the national sport of Thailand. I decided to join. Six months later, I was in the ring.

When I was twenty years old, my parents asked me if I would like to have a big party for my twenty-first birthday. I told them I would rather go to Thailand to learn the art of Muay Thai. I spent three months

1

there training with the world's best Muay Thai fighters. By the time I returned home, I was a year older and a better fighter by several levels.

The following year I competed for my national colors. My great friend and training partner would also compete. We were told the night before the bout that we were going to fight each other. He nearly knocked me down in the first twenty seconds, hitting me with a straight punch to the face. My head was ringing, and I had the taste of metal in my mouth. I got up, shaking my head, on the verge of quitting. Something happened. We fought for the full four rounds. He is a tough opponent, and as a boxer, he is known as "The Pitbull." He has a boxing history and a heavy hand. We trained together twice every day. He made me tough and taught me how to take a strike. It's easy to throw a strike, but taking one is a different story. It was a bit of a surreal experience.

As the fight progressed, I gained more confidence and belief in my ability. I stuck to the basics: chin down, hands up. I got stronger and stronger through the fight and finally won on points. It was a key moment in my fighting career because I was on the brink of giving up, but then something stirred in my heart. I thought of my family and those I love, and I fought well and won against the odds. I was the 2007 national lightweight Muay Thai champion. This was quite an awesome stage of my life, because I rose through the ranks quickly. I was a senior student at the University of Cape Town at the time and in my final year of studying, as well as teaching private students and group classes at Dragon Power gym. It was a balancing act, and I was succeeding. At this stage I had completed five fights with no losses.

Later that year we flew up from the corner of Africa for the International Federation of Muay Thai Amateurs (IFMA) world championship that was held in Bangkok. It's the only tournament of its kind, with many countries represented from all over the world. It's a knockout tournament, so you need to win to progress through. As an amateur tournament, it consists of four rounds of two minutes, with a one-minute break. Fighters must wear leg pads, head guards, chest guards, elbow guards, gloves, and mouth and groin protection. Eight minutes may sound like a short time, but it is intense! It's a totally different style of fighting, because the time limit is so short. The extra safety padding adds to the intensity, giving you more protection, which means you strike more frequently and keep doing so right until the end. If your opponent hits you once, you must hit him or her twice. The chest guards constrict your breathing as you gasp for air more and more intensely through the fight. The head guard gives you tunnel vision, and shin and elbow guards are to give you added weight.

The bus trip to the shopping mall, where the tournament was being held, took about two hours. I remember listening to Radiohead and doing as I always do before a fight—thinking of my family and past experiences. My first fight was against Portugal. I was still an inexperienced fighter, and the nerves were immense. I destroyed Portugal in forty seconds in the first round. A few knees to the head, and the referee stopped the fight. Awesome—I got through to the next round. The next day was a totally different fight than before; I was to fight the United States. We battled through the rounds. We threw each other down and kicked and punched nonstop. It was really close, and by the end of the fight, we were exhausted. We had pushed ourselves beyond our limits. I won on points. I had injured my leg from all the kicking and blocking. It was black and blue all over, and I had to lie down and put ice on it directly after the fight. I made it to the semifinal against Ukraine the following day. Fortunately my injury was just severe bruising, so I could still fight. Every morning we had to weigh in and were inspected by a doctor. I was pretty nervous about him seeing my leg, but he was more concerned about my thumb, which had ballooned after my fight with Portugal. All was good. In the space of three days, I had progressed more as a fighter than at any previous point during my fighting career. It becomes a campaign. Now I was into the stages where, whatever happened, I would get a medal for my achievements. The first thing I did when the fight started was throw a strike with my injured leg, to force myself to work through the injury. When you fight, you don't really feel pain unless it's serious—the rush of the fight takes the pain away. It was another intense battle, where it took everything I had to get through the rounds. It was clear he had more experience than me, switching stances with ease and throwing spinning back

punches (which I started practicing as soon as I was back in the gym).
I managed to throw him down a couple of times, and I was always on
my front foot. Toward the end of the fight, I also switched my stance,
which I had never done before, and ducked under a body kick in the
last few seconds (which I had also never done before). The bell rang
for the final round. I grabbed our South African flag and wrapped it
around my body and waved it in the air. The South African coaches,
team, and my family were cheering and were a great support. Decision
time. The referee raised my opponent's hand. I was devastated. I
thought I had done enough to win the fight, but this is life—some you
win, and some you lose. It was my first loss and also a big learning process for me. Nevertheless, it was a successful campaign, and I was voted
South Africa's best male fighter. It is true that you do learn more from
a defeat than from a victory. It's a time for self-refection, and doubt in
your ability may creep in. It's the perfect time to get back into the gym
and into the ring to improve yourself.

It was now 2008. At this stage, I had completed my degree and
stayed in Cape Town. I was given a job as a store manager at a popular
local bakery after striking up a conversation with my friend's father,
who was the owner, and he gave me the opportunity. I continued training, teaching, and fighting, as well as putting in the hours in the work-
place. I was up at 5:00 a.m. and sometimes arrived home as late as 9:00
p.m. It was a challenging time, and I was burning myself out, despite
the great support my girlfriend and family were giving me. I had to
think hard about what I wanted, and eventually I resigned from my
job, as I told them I wanted to get a gold medal at the world championships. I won my national colors again, and this time the team was
headed for Busan in South Korea, where the IFMA tournament was to
be held that year.

Korea was a somewhat similar experience to the previous year,
although now I had a more powerful belief system and knew what I
could achieve. I beat Japan on points in a not-too-exciting fight; I just
bullied my way through. The same happened against China. This time
I was in the final against Iran. Again I had three fights in three days.
Iran was an awesome fighter. We fought toe-to-toe in the first round

before he knocked me down with a head kick at the end of the round. I got up and recovered, but I was shaken. We continued our battle into the second round. Another head kick, and he knocked me out cold. Damn! So close to winning the gold medal, but I got the silver.

I currently have the amateur fight record of thirteen wins from sixteen fights. I have taught for years, opened my own school in the past, and still teach and train for the fun of it. I'm by no means the best fighter to have walked the earth, but I have earned a wealth of knowledge from this martial art and have some tips for any aspiring martial artist, or anyone at all. The rules and values of martial arts can be applied to pretty much anything.

two

Values

I will begin by sharing with you the values of Muay Thai and how they are applied inside and outside the ring.

Discipline

To be successful in the ring, it is absolutely necessary to be disciplined in your training. You need to be on time every training day and in possession of all your training equipment, so you can spend the allotted time for training. It is not normal for a human being to watch someone while he or she is being attacked. You have to discipline your mind to watch attacks, to overcome your natural aversion to seeing attacks, and to learn from what you see. Training consistently in the mornings and evenings is one of the toughest challenges, but it is essential for progression.

Commitment

This runs parallel with discipline. A fighter has to commit to his or her training program, trainers, and training partners. It can be tough not only for the fighters but also for their loved ones, as a lot of energy (seen and unseen) has to be put into training and fighting. Fortunately this spent energy is repaid and has a positive effect on other areas of the fighter's life.

Belief

This is one of my favorite elements of fighting. Fighters have to believe in themselves and what they are doing. A strong belief system has to be cultivated to be an accomplished fighter. You must go into the ring believing you will win.

Respect

This is the most important value of fighting. A fighter has to have respect. In Muay Thai, there is a dance we do before the fight called the Wai Kru, which means showing respect to the teacher. You bow to your opponent before you fight and again afterward. You respect each other as fighters and as martial artists, since you both respect Muay Thai as an art form.

three

Muay Thai

As mentioned, you have eight weapons in Muay Thai: boxing, kicking, elbows, and knees. Kicks and punches are generally used for longer-range striking, while knees and elbows are used at close range. The principle is that you stay calm and focused and breathe consistently, but when you strike, you hit with maximum force.

As you progress, you will learn to add various combinations and use different strikes together. Just remember that this is the most brutal ring sport, and it is also an art form, so it will take time for you to progress. Remember to focus on the basics. Breathe, and everything else will come. Also remember to protect yourself at all costs. Keep your guard up and your chin down, move around effectively, and try to put yourself into your opponent's mind, so you can stay a step ahead. Boxing is a great form to use as an attack; you can use your jab to keep your opponent at bay. Remember that Muay Thai boxing is different from regular boxing in that we use a different stance. Muay Thai kicking is renowned as extremely dangerous, because we kick our opponents with the bones of our shins. We also drive forward with the hips and kick through the opponent for maximum effectiveness.

Elbows are devastating. Sometimes being hit with a boxing strike can feel like being hit by a rock—now imagine being hit with the tiny tip of an elbow! Using your elbows is a quick way to end a fight, because it often draws blood, so the fight will be stopped. Knees are great to use when you are in close and when you are holding and manipulating your opponent in the grapple. Of course, a knee to the head will most likely end a fight, so if possible you should aim to pull your opponent's head down toward the knee and strike him or her.

On the defensive side, always keep upright in the grapple to avoid being pulled down. This brings me into the grapple, or clinch, which can be considered a ninth weapon. Quite often, large portions of fights will be spent in the grapple. Remember to keep calm. Being so close to your opponent may cause you to struggle or be anxious. Keep breathing. Try to get into effective positions, where you can throw your elbows and knees and ultimately take your opponent to the ground. Muay Thai is about balance. You have to strike with maximum force, and stay calm and breathe, so remember that composure is extremely important. It's not just a fight; it's also a mental game. Another important thing to remember is to have fun. You are participating in an ancient art form that is benefitting your body and your mind. Your body will be encouraged to become its ideal weight, with a focus on core strength. Not too light, and not too heavy, but lean and strong— exactly what most of us want! Most of my students have, in fact, been women, as they want to train to get their bodies in shape. In this world, where our minds are constantly worried about the future or what has happened in the past, Muay Thai will bring you into the present moment, and you will feel the mental benefits and elevation of mood. There is also a big endorphin rush, so the psychological benefits are great. Enjoy the transformation process; it's an incredible experience! Now I'll show you how to do it.

four

Techniques

The Basic Stance

Put your feet together, and raise your hands in the air. Clench both fists, keeping the thumbs on the outside of your fingers. Drop your hands, and place the right hand at the back of the jaw, beside the ear, and the left hand in front of your face. Keep your wrists pointing straight up, nice and tight, elbows in, and shoulders relaxed.

Take a short step out with your left leg, with a forty-five-degree angle between the left side and straight in front of you. Keep your back heel off the ground. Your left leg should be pointing straight in front of you, and your right leg should be pointing forty-five degrees between the right and straight in front of you. Visualize an opponent in front of you. Your shoulders must be square, and there should be a gap between your legs, so that if you visualized two lines, they would be parallel to each other. It's important to keep your body square to your opponent for power, and it's important to keep the parallel gap between your legs for balance. Now that you are in position, you must shift your weight from one leg to the other. Just lift one leg slightly, then put it to the ground, and lift the other, and continue with this motion. Do not swing your hips back and forward; just lift each leg slightly back and forward. Don't rush—it's a controlled movement, and there is no need to hop from one foot to the other. It's called the 50/50 stance, which means you are always shifting your weight 50 percent on one and then 50 percent on the other. You should never be flat-footed, and this stance ensures that you are always ready to attack, defend, or counterattack. One of the most important rules of fighting is to dip your chin, and keep it down. The other most important rule is to keep your hands up. You must protect yourself. With your chin down and your hands up, you are safe from strikes to the face. With your shoulders relaxed and elbows in, you are protecting your torso, and with the 50/50 stance, your legs are always ready for action. Remember that everything can be done in reverse if you are southpaw (right leg in front).

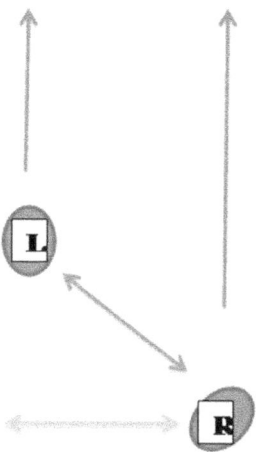

The figure above shows how your feet should be positioned in the 50/50 stance, with the left leg in the front and the right at the back. The blue lines show that, in the stance, you must keep a gap between your legs. This is further illustrated by the red line. Never have one foot behind the other—you need to keep this gap for balance. The orange line shows how your shoulders are square and not at an angle. The right foot is at a forty-five-degree angle. When you move in this stance, whichever direction you step in, you need to lead with the foot closest to that direction. For example, if you step forward, you need to step forward with your front foot; the back foot will come forward naturally. If you step to the left, you step first with your left foot, and if you step to the right, you must step first with the right foot. This enables you to keep the gap between your legs and so maintain balance. Keep your eyes fixed on your opponent's chest area. Don't look at him or her in the eyes, as this may bring unnecessary emotion to your fight. By focusing on the chest area, you will also begin training your peripheral vision, which is an essential part of fighting. Your peripheral vision allows you to see what you are not looking at directly, so by looking at the chest area, you will be able to see any strike that is coming your way. Muay Thai is controlled and smooth in this stance, but when you strike, you give it 100 percent, so here we go.

Punching

Punches are great for attack and counterattack. They can be done quickly and require less energy than kicking. Look for gaps in your opponent's guard. Use your jab frequently to keep your opponent at bay and to check your distance. Use combinations to throw your opponent off guard and set yourself up to strike him or her effectively. Use body shots when up close, but always keep an eye out for a clear strike to the head. If your opponent is attacking you, use punches as a form of defense, and launch a counterattack.

Jab: The jab is a straight strike with the front hand, so if you are standing in the regular stance, it will be your left hand that strikes. From the 50/50 stance, you need to initiate the move by taking a short, quick step forward with your left leg. While you are doing this, you must begin to rotate your shoulders in a clockwise direction (if you are looking down on the position from above). As with everything in Muay Thai, it's not the forward-moving motion that gives you power but rather the rotating action of your core. It's all about the core. Keeping your hand at eye level, start punching forward, and rotate the wrist straight, so your knuckles will be hitting your opponent. By twisting the wrist straight, you can force your elbow to rise up and get in line with the wrist, giving you maximum power. Once you have thrown the jab, pull the wrist, and rotate your shoulders back into position. Use your jab on attack and defense. It's a good way to keep your opponent away and check the distance between you. You can also be devastating on attack when you spot a gap between your opponent's hands and take the opportunity to strike his or her face.

Cross: The cross punch is similar to the jab but is a straight strike with the back hand. You initiate the move by taking a short step forward with your left leg. You need to bring your left hand back to your face at eye level, pressing it against your head. Strike forward with the right hand, and turn your wrist so your knuckles are parallel to the floor. This will bring your elbow up so your arm is in a straight line when you strike. Remember that you must rotate your core and shoulders counterclockwise. The left hand must stay up to keep you protected while you strike.

1-2 (One-Two): This is a combination of the jab and the cross punch, done in one motion. Don't rush the movements; make sure your technique is sound. First, strike with a jab, then bring the left hand back to the face, rotate your core the other way, and strike with the right hand. It's as simple as that. One thing I notice often with beginners is that they drop the hand they are not striking with. Make sure you keep your hands at eye level all the time. Make sure that whichever hand is not striking is held high, right against your face. If either of your hands drops while striking, you will open up opportunities for your opponent to counterattack, and this could lose you the fight.

Hook: Hooks need to be done from a very close range to be effective. A hook needs to come from the side and hit your opponent at the side of his or her face or body, so you need to be pretty close. To do this, you need to give yourself room with the hand you are striking with. This does pose an element of risk, because you will expose yourself for a short time. Initiate the move with a short step forward. Move your left hand forward and away from you, and lift your elbow so that it's parallel to the floor. Now rotate your core clockwise, and strike with your hand to the side of your opponent's head. All the same applies to the right hand—just remember to bring your left hand back, and keep it up. Your shoulders provide power, so for extra power, rotate the shoulder in the same direction as your strike. The hook is very good on counterattack; if you block an opponent's punch, his or her face will be vulnerable on the side that he or she strikes with, and you could immediately counter with a hook. Hooks are dangerous weapons, and because they are done from close up, they are powerful. They can hurt you even if you are blocking. Hooks to the body can also do damage, so look for gaps in your opponent's defense, and aim for the rib area (a strike here can also wind your opponent, making it hard for him or her to breathe, which is exactly what you want in a fight!) The reality is, however, that Muay Thai fighters have extremely well-conditioned bodies, and it will take a good strike to knock the wind out of your opponent.

Uppercut: Similar to the hook, the uppercut is generally done from a close distance. The best target to strike with the uppercut would be underneath the chin of your opponent. Uppercuts are generally not that easy to land, so timing and patience are critical elements. As with the hook, there is an element of risk involved due to exposing your face on the side that you are striking with. Initiate the move by taking a short step forward. Drop your left hand in a circular motion, down and toward your body slightly, and then rotate up and away toward the underside of your opponent's chin. When you strike, your fist should be facing straight up. As with the hook, the shoulder can provide extra power, so rotate your shoulder in the same circular motion as your arm. When you initiate the move, tilt the body down on the left side, and tilt it back straight when you strike. Apply the same movement, but in reverse for the right hand, keeping the left hand up close against your chin. When you are close to your opponent, look for opportunities to uppercut his or her chin.

Blocking: It's really simple to block against a boxing attack. Bring your left hand back, and press the knuckles against the top of your head so that your right and left hand are pressed against your forehead. Keep your elbows in to protect the body. In this position, you are very well protected. Just remember, you are not a punching bag, so rather than standing there and taking the strikes, get back into a position where you can attack.

Kicking

Thais are renowned for their devastating roundhouse kicks, and if you go to Thailand and train, you will see why. They kick, kick, and kick some more! It's important that when you throw your kick, you give it maximum power, maximum speed, lead with the hip, and kick *through* your opponent. By kicking through your opponent, I mean that you should not be aiming to stop your kick when at the point of contact, but aim to kick right through your opponent, which means you will give a more devastating strike.

Teep: This is a straight strike with your leg, also known as a push kick. For a kick from the left front leg, you must keep your right foot firmly on the ground (heel on the ground). Give yourself a firm footing on the right leg, and keep it strong; this provides the basis of your strength. Lift your left leg straight toward your opponent, and tilt your body slightly back. Extend the leg and hips forward, striking at the core of your opponent. Your leg should be only slightly bent. You need to strike quickly to avoid your opponent anticipating the move. Although it is known as a push kick, you must strike as if it were a punch with 100-percent power. Teeps can be devastating; they can wind your opponent or knock him or her off balance. They also can be done to the legs (although not directly on the knee) and to the face, but this requires greater accuracy than if striking at the core area. Teep kicks are extremely good for keeping your opponent away from you.

Roundhouse: The roundhouse kick must be done with explosive power and practiced until it becomes second nature. The left leg is a little tricky. At the beginner level, initiate the move by taking a short step up and slightly out with the right foot. Once this is done, launch your left leg up, and bring it around to the side of your opponent. It's important that you don't kick up. The hip must lead the movement, so when you hit your opponent, your leg and hips are facing in toward your opponent and not up. Imagine your leg is a log, and you are swinging it through with your hips. It's not a flick—you must visualize yourself kicking all the way through your opponent, leading with your hips. A better way to do the front roundhouse kick (and you should keep practicing until this becomes second nature) is to initiate the strike with a switch step. This means you do a short hop, and switch your left leg to the back and the right leg to the front, and from there you launch your left-leg kick toward your opponent. The initial movement is up but then turns sideways. The back kick is slightly different. As your left leg is pointing straight forward, you need to take a short step, slightly out and forward, and open the foot so that it is turned around forty-five degrees from the straight position. This will force your hip to come through at a horizontal position when you kick your opponent. Once you have perfected this practice of coming up onto your toes when you strike, your kicks will have more power. For your right leg, take a short step forward with your left foot. This time, when you step, turn your foot out, so it's pointing forty-five degrees toward the left side. This will allow the hips to come through so you kick properly; do everything the same as with your left leg. Remember to return to your stance after the kick. You can strike roundhouse kicks at your opponent's legs, torso, or head.

Blocking: Blocking against kicks is extremely important. If you don't block against kicks, you will not last. Kicks to the legs can do damage to the muscles, which will cause discomfort and make movement difficult and possibly end the fight. Kicks to the ribs can break them, and kicks to the head will most likely cause a knockout. (I have personal experience of this—keep your hands up!) To block against a kick, all you need to do is lift the leg on the same side that your opponent is kicking. So, if your opponent were kicking with the right leg, you would lift your left leg. Lift the left leg out at forty-five degrees, and bring it up high toward your elbow. Don't hit the leg on your elbow; keep your elbow on the outside, pressing against the leg. For your right leg, all you need to do is lift it, as it is already at an outside angle. When you block, keep your leg relaxed—don't tighten your muscles. You are hitting bone against bone, so you must keep your leg relaxed to absorb the kick. Balance is critical here, because you are standing on one leg. Make sure the leg you are standing on is strong. Practice blocking until it becomes second nature. Once you have blocked a kick, you have not only defended yourself but also set yourself up for a good opportunity to counterattack.

Elbows

Elbows were taken out of some forms of fighting, because they are considered deadly weapons. Being hit with a glove can feel like being hit with a rock, but an elbow can be even more potent. Lift your elbow straight up until it's in line with your shoulder, and pull your wrist back toward your shoulder. Feel the tip of your elbow as it points forward. Compare that tiny tip with the surface area of a glove, and you can imagine what kind of damage the elbow can do to your opponent. Elbows can be difficult to land effectively, though, so timing and opportunity are key elements to making them work. You have to be close to your opponent to land an elbow.

Straight elbow: Step forward with your left leg. Keeping your guard up, bring your left elbow up, and tuck your arm in as tightly as possible. As you bring it up, turn it out away from your body, so when you strike, your elbow will cut across your opponent's face. Rotate your core as you do the strike. Try to focus on bringing your elbow up and coming down across your opponent's face. The right elbow is done with the same technique; just ensure that your left hand is up, protecting your face.

Up elbow: This must be done quickly when you see a gap to strike your opponent's chin, similar to an uppercut. Take a short step forward, tuck the left arm in so your elbow is sharp, rotate your core, and strike with the point of your elbow onto your opponent's chin in an upward motion. Do the same for your right elbow. Keep it tight, and keep your hands close to your head. Your opponent must not see this one coming.

Down elbow: Initiate this by taking a short step forward. Tuck in your left arm and rotate your elbow back behind your body, then up, and strike down onto your opponent's face. While you are doing this, rotate your core. Do the same for your right elbow.

Knees

Knees, like elbows, also have to be done at close range. Knees are extremely powerful and also show good technique and can win you points in a fight. A knee to the head is almost guaranteed to end things, but knees can be effective also when striking the torso and legs.

Straight knee: Initiate the strike with a step forward. Grab around your opponent's neck, leading with the front hand first. Tuck your leg in, like you do with your arm with the elbow strike, pull your opponent toward your knee, and thrust your knee forward. Drive forward with the hip, and tilt the body slightly backward for extra power. When you have the hang of it, try coming up onto your toes when you strike. Most knees are thrown when in the clinch (or grapple), which we will discuss later.

Side knee: When you strike with the knee, you also can strike from the side, like with a roundhouse kick. Step forward, tighten the knee in, and bring it up and out before bringing it in toward your opponent, striking in the rib area or the side of the leg. When you are in the clinch, practice initiating the move with a short hop with the opposite leg in the same outward direction in which your knee is moving. This would mean that, for the left knee, you push off of the left foot and land with your right foot where your left foot was, while kicking your left leg out and then bringing it in for the knee strike to your opponent. It is important to kick your leg out far and then curl your knee in tight and throw the strike. This shows good technique, will get you points in the ring, and will do more damage to your opponent. Only do this if you are in the clinch position, though, so you can use your opponent for balance.

Grappling (Clinch)

We often say that there are eight weapons in Muay Thai. There is a ninth, however: grappling. This is when you are in close and holding your opponent, and he or she holds you, as you work for positions to strike or throw your opponent to the ground. A large amount of your time is spent grappling, so it must be practiced in order to master the art.

The basics: The basic stance involves having your left hand behind your opponent's neck, pulling down and toward yourself. The right hand holds your opponent's left arm, pulling down. Your opponent would be in the same position. It's extremely important to remember that as soon as you come into the grapple, your mind-set should shift into grappling mode. You must keep your chin up. This is because if you keep your chin down, as you do when you are fighting, your opponent will easily be able to pull your head down from behind your neck. From there he or she easily can strike a knee to your head. I don't need to say more. So, get high up onto your toes, and keep your chin up. Feel your opponent's body and the way he or she is moving. You don't necessarily have to have either leg forward in the grapple. Stay on your toes, and move your feet to balance yourself accordingly. You are holding on to your opponent; this provides you with balance and allows you to throw knees easily. Many people make the mistake of overexerting during the grapple, getting tired and losing their form, which leaves them vulnerable. In the grapple, you should be gaining your breath and your strength. Stay composed; use your own body weight to manipulate your opponent. You can even just hang on to your opponent to wear him or her down. This is especially effective if you feel your opponent overexerting and trying to force things. Make him or her tired. Wear him or her down slowly. Use your body weight by leaning backward and pulling backward toward you instead of pushing against your opponent. The best position in the grapple is to have both hands on the inside, behind your opponent's neck, in order to put maximum downward pressure and bring his or her head down, exposing him or her to potential head strikes with the knee. When you have this inside grip, you also have maximum control over the body and can shift him or her more easily into your desired position. From the basic stance, with your left hand already behind your opponent's neck, you need to quickly drop the right hand underneath your opponent's left arm and bring it behind the neck. Now you have both hands behind your opponent's neck. Remember to lock them strongly behind the neck, and try to pull the head down using your own body weight, tilting the hands downward. Your opponent will try to do the same thing—getting both hands behind your neck—so it becomes a kind of dance as you both move your hands inside. Remember to move quickly when you go for the inside, as you expose yourself very briefly to elbow strikes. Don't go for the inside with both hands at the same time, because then you completely expose yourself. Don't be scared to pull your opponent close to you, limiting both your opponent's and your own movements. When you have the grip behind the head, pull the neck down, and, while doing that, dig your elbow into his or her shoulder with the same arm, causing him or her discomfort. Try to aggravate your opponent to get him or her to overexert. Use your body weight, keep calm, and breathe. Naturally, being so close to your opponent may make you scared and more willing to use all your force to beat him or her. Do the opposite. Wait for the right moment to strike. Throw your side knees to get points, using your opponent's body weight for balance. Wait for his or her hand to drop, and then throw your elbow. Keep your hands inside. When he or she tries to come inside, turn your elbow in to make it more difficult for your opponent, which can cause him or her to keep the outside grip. When he or she grabs you behind your head, close the shoulder, bringing the chin close to the shoulder. This will make it difficult for him or her to lock behind your neck and will cause discomfort on your opponent's wrist.

Taking your opponent to the ground: Being able to get your opponent on the ground shows that you have excellent technical skills and will get you points in a fight. It can also be very demoralizing for your opponent to be thrown to the ground and can assist in breaking his or her spirit. In Thailand I learned a simple but effective way to bring your opponent to the ground. As a lightweight, I can bring even the biggest fighters to the ground easily using this simple method. In the grapple, wait for your opponent to strike with a knee. If your opponent strikes with the left knee, then you will have to use your left hand, and vice versa. Make sure the hand is inside, gripping the back of the neck. As your opponent strikes, pull on the back of the head with your hand, and push your hips forward into your opponent's. Pull back and away from your body, bringing your opponent past the left side of your body if you're using your left hand. Lean back, and use your body weight to do this. Your opponent is only standing on one leg, so he or she will fall easily down at your side. Make sure your left leg is pressed close to his or her stabilizing right leg, so that he or she can't hop on it for balance. Timing is the critical element here. Throw knees, which will encourage your opponent to do the same. As you are in the grapple and really close, your opponent won't be able to see your eyes, so you can watch his or her legs and wait for the right moment. You also can fall on top of your opponent when you do this, which can wind him or her and drain more of his or her energy. This can be very demoralizing. When you throw your opponent to the ground, keep holding him or her, turning so he or she is underneath you. Then fall with your opponent, and land on top of him or her.

five

Top Tips

Always keep your hands up. Keep your chin down, except in the grapple. Always watch your opponent unless you are doing an advanced technique that requires you to momentarily turn your eyes away. When your opponent takes his or her eyes off you, it's a sign that his or her spirit is broken, and you should be able to win the fight. Keep your shoulders relaxed and your elbows in. Keep your wrists tight. Strike with maximum power, but stay focused between strikes. My students sometimes joke with me about how often I tell them to breathe during class, but it's so important. You must learn how to breathe effectively and how to control your breathing. This will be one of your great strengths and keep you going at maximum efficiency in a fight. When you strike, make sure you make a noise. It can be a short hiss or a growl or a howl, but make sure to make a noise as you hit. This encourages you to breathe. When you are running low on air, slow down and take a few deep breaths. Don't concern yourself too much over what will happen in the ring—focus on the things you can control: your training, fitness, technique, and a positive mind-set. Visualize what will happen in the ring. It will surprise you how often what you visualize comes to fruition in the ring. Don't undervalue what you can do; you may surprise yourself. It is you against another fighter. You both have the same weapons, so the playing field is even. Be confident, and show this confidence to the judges and to your opponent. Do the Wai Kru with pride, and walk in the ring like you are the boss. It shows you have no fear. Think of where you come from, your family, and how you have come to be in the ring. Think of all the long hours of training and dedication, and think of those you love—all of these will give you strength. You are there for a reason, and you'll compete as best you can, win or lose.

six

Benefits of Fighting

Fighting and training in Muay Thai is all about breaking the limitations that you have put on yourself. You'll find that you can push harder and go further than you imagined. The learning is continuous, and you will always improve. This is what makes it so addictive. Your body will change, your core will become strong, and you will move toward being your ideal weight. You will eat more healthily, as your body tells you what it needs for the energy it is using. You don't have to be a fighter to enjoy the benefits of Muay Thai. Being the world's most brutal ring sport, it is excellent for self-defense. You can do it for weight loss, fitness, or simply for the fun of it. Muay Thai takes the mind out of the past and the future and puts it in the present moment. It takes you out of the world you are in, and when you come out, you feel amazing. Your body has worked hard, and your mind has let go. It can be enjoyed by almost all. It's even great for kids, both physically and mentally, because they have to work hard and focus but can also have fun.

seven

Teamwork

As with anything in life, it is important to surround yourself with people you can share energy with and to push each other to higher levels. Your coach, training partners, support network, and your corner are the people who will enable you to compete as best you can. We all know that getting to the gym can be difficult, because we usually have so many things going on in our lives. If you know there is someone who will meet you there and train with you, it makes the job easier and more fun, and you will learn more quickly. Find training partners, and set up your training regime. Mix it up with morning runs, evening sparring sessions, and weight training, and schedule the times in your diary. It's extremely stimulating and fun when you start planning what days and times you will be training and also what training you will do and with whom. Different people have different strengths in different areas, so try to feed off that to make you the most accomplished fighter you can be. For example, if you know that someone is a great grappler, set up a time with him or her for a grappling session. Or if you know a good runner, set up a time to have a run with him or her. This will benefit your training and will also help you network with like-minded individuals who will support you inside and outside the ring.

eight

Training

The bulk of your training should be martial arts training at your gym. It is best to train barefoot, and the floor should be padded. Skipping is a great way to warm up and teaches you to stay on your toes, breathe consistently, and keep your elbows in and shoulders relaxed, which are all critical elements in fighting. Shadowboxing is extremely important and is also a great way to warm up. Shadowboxing allows you to practice and refine your techniques, but it also lets you visualize and get into the right mind-set.

Pad work is one of the most important parts of your training. You partner up, and one person puts on kick pads (pads that extend to the elbow so you can punch and kick), and you put on your gloves. Holding pads is an art in itself. You learn about fighting when you strike pads. Set the time, such as four rounds of three minutes, and then go for it. A good pad holder will make you work on all your techniques and push you to go hard. When you strike pads, you can unleash and strike with maximum power. Focus on your breathing. This will help you strike as hard and fast as possible but also will allow you to keep in control and stop you from passing out. It's a balancing act. Remember when you strike to make a sound and go hard, but when you are not striking, breathe, keep your guard up, chin down, and watch. Your pad holder should strike with the pads if you drop your hands and kick you to get you to block. This makes it more realistic and gets you to work on your defense. He or she should be wearing leg pads so he or she can kick you at any time without hurting you. When you do pads, focus on all elements of striking and defensive work (punches, kicks, elbows, and knees). Make sure you push yourself to the max in the last few moments of your last round. Go for combos and repetition. Doing ten kicks in a row with the same leg will get your kicks stronger and force you to breathe properly.

Sparring is obviously a key element of your training. It can be quite daunting, but just keep practicing, and you'll improve and grow in confidence. This is the closest you get to the real thing, and sparring can be such fun. This is the time where you actually start to learn to take a strike. It's easy to throw a punch, but taking one is harder. Just focus on the basics, and try to outsmart your opponent. Move around, and learn how to control your space. Don't allow your partner to over-whelm you—look for ways to exploit and attack.

Bag work is also fun and versatile. Try and find the larger, heavier, bags for your training, as they will offer you more resistance and give you better conditioning. You can push yourself with the bag and work your cardio, or you can use it to practice and refine your technique. The bag doesn't hit you back, which also means you can focus on exactly what you want to do. When you strike the bag, make sure you don't try and push the bag when you make contact. Hit hard, but pull back after your strike.

Outside of your martial arts training, you should run. Put some shoes on, and hit the road. It gets oxygen into the body, makes the legs strong, increases lung capacity, and clears the mind. Pushing weights are good for strength and power. Find your own balance with your training regimen.

nine

Training Gear

Muay Thai is a cheap sport to participate in. Here is a list of items you should buy and take with you to your gym.

- Boxing gloves—ten-ounce gloves are usually the preferred size
- Boxing wraps (always wrap your hands before you don your gloves; they support and protect the wrists, fingers, and knuckles)
- Skipping rope
- Mouth guard
- Head guard
- Leg pads (for sparring)
- Kick pads (pads that strap onto the arms that extend to the elbows)
- Groin guard

ten

Before the Bell

I hope this handbook adds value to any aspiring fighter or anyone training in the art of Muay Thai. The techniques, methods, and tips have been tried and tested. I also hope the book inspires those who have not tried Muay Thai to take it up. Take the first step—you won't regret it.